Paleo Recipes
Delicious Mexican Style Recipes!

Contents

About the Book

This book is health conscious people following the Paleo diet who love Mexican style food. You may get a better understanding about the Paleo diet and its health benefits within the Introduction. This book comprises a collection of recipes for every meal of the day. Start your day with healthy and delicious breakfast recipes including muffins, frittatas, sausage, breakfast bars, egg dishes and lots more. Following breakfast, are lunch recipes that are light and delicious. Then comes the most important meal of the day "dinner". The spicy dinner recipes include salsa, soup, poultry and fish. Lastly, indulge your sweet tooth without even breaking the rules! Enjoy the collection of delicious and nutritious recipes while getting into your new habits.

Introduction

The Paleolithic diet is a way of eating from 10,000 years ago in the Paleolithic era, also known as the caveman diet, Stone Age diet and hunter gathered diet. The Paleo diet consists of foods that were eaten before the agricultural revolution and wheat based diet. These diets consist of meat, seafood, fruits, vegetables and nuts. All foods in their natural form, not processed and wheat free are included. Studies are showing that human bodies are better adapted to this way of eating.

Foods in their natural form contain a great deal of vitamins and minerals. By including these in daily eating, many health benefits may be achieved. Following the Paleo diet, people have reclaimed a healthy body weight, lowered cholesterol, decreased high blood pressure, decreased cardiac problems, experienced increased energy and stabilized blood sugar levels. Many of the traditional recipes that people love, have a Paleo version that are just as delicious, if not more so. An added bonus is you are giving your body the nutrients it needs, so there is no guilt. Best of luck on your journey eating clean with Paleo! These recipes can be a starting point to help you create new favorite meals.

Breakfast

Banana Nut Chocolate Chip Muffins

3-4 Servings

2 bananas

1½ cup almond flour

1 tsp. baking soda

1 tsp. baking powder

1 tsp. cinnamon

1 tsp. vanilla

2 eggs (whisked)

1/4 c. coconut oil (melted)

1/3 c. walnuts or pecans

1 to 2 tbsp. raw honey

1/2 c. mini chocolate chips

Pinch of salt

Take a small bowl and smash the bananas. Add eggs, coconut oil, vanilla and honey, blend them together. Now take a large bowl, add baking powder, almond flour, baking soda, cinnamon & salt, mix them well. Add the small bowl mixture into the large bowl and blend well. Add half the chopped nuts and chocolate chips, blend well. Pour it into silicone muffin cups. Sprinkle with remaining nuts on top of muffins. Bake it in oven at 350 degrees for 22 to 25 minutes. Serve warm or store in refrigerator.

Prosciutto Wrapped Asparagus

2-4 Servings

8 slices prosciutto (ingredients should be ham & salt only)

16 spears fresh asparagus

Vegetable oil or coconut oil

Rinse & dry the asparagus spears and break off the hard ends. Cut the prosciutto lengthwise in half. Wrap the prosciutto around asparagus spears from bottom towards top. Don't cover completely. Take a skillet and heat some oil and fry asparagus on medium high heat for 3 minutes on both sides. Prosciutto wrapped asparagus is now ready to serve.

Paleo Breakfast Porridge

2-4 Servings

2 bananas (mashed)

2 c. coconut milk

3/4 c. almond meal

1/4 c. flax meal

1 tsp. cinnamon

1 tsp. ginger

1/8 tsp. ground cloves

1/8 tsp. ground nutmeg

1/8 tsp. sea salt

Raw honey (optional)

Berries, unsweetened coconut flakes, nuts etc. (optional)

Take a medium sized saucepan and combine all the ingredients. Warm it on medium high heat until it boils. Stir until thick and bubbly.

Mexican Rice Bowls

3-4 Servings

1 head of cauliflower (cut into florets)

1/3 c. water or broth

1 tsp. garlic powder

1/8 tsp. cayenne pepper

2 tsp. lime juice

1/2 lb. pork chorizo

1/2 lb. ground beef

1/2 white onion (diced)

1 avocado (diced)

Salsa of choice

Some fresh cilantro (roughly chopped)

Salt and pepper (to taste)

Take a food processor or use a grater to made small pieces of cauliflower. Add cauliflower, water or broth and some salt in a small saucepan. Keep it covered on over medium heat and let it steam for about 10 minutes. Stir it to avoid sticking to the bottom. When cauliflower becomes soft, add garlic powder, cilantro, lime, cayenne pepper, and a bit of salt and pepper. While rice is cooking, place a medium skillet over medium-high heat and cook chorizo and ground beef. Divide into small pieces & cook until cooked completely. When cauliflower rice and meat are ready to cook, add rice, onion, avocado, meat, and salsa to a bowl.

Tomato Basil Frittata

4-6 Servings

10 large eggs

5 bacon slices (cut into small chunks)

1 large red onion (thinly slice)

4 oz. baby spinach leaves

2 small tomatoes (thinly sliced)

3 tsp. wholegrain or homemade mustard

Fresh basil leaves (for garnishing)

1 tbsp. Paleo cooking fat or clarified butter

Sea salt (to taste)

Freshly ground black pepper (to taste)

Pre-heat the oven to 350 F. Beat the eggs and mustard in a bowl and season to taste. Heat up the cooking fat in a skillet over a medium heat; add bacon and onion to cook for 5 to 6 minutes or until golden. Put spinach leaves into the skillet and cook for 1 to 2 minutes or until the spinach wilts. Shift the egg mixture into the skillet; cook until it stiffens and arrange the tomatoes on top. When the frittata is set around the edges, place the skillet into the oven and bake for 30 minutes or until turns to a nice golden color. Shake some basil leaves on top and serve.

Green Chili Omelet

3 Servings

6 eggs

1/2 tsp. salt

1/4 tsp. pepper

2 tbsp. green chilies (chopped)

1 tbsp. butter

In a small bowl beat salt and pepper with eggs and stir in chilies. Take a skillet, thaw butter on medium heat and add half egg mixture. Let the eggs stiffen. Once eggs fully set, remove them from heat. Fold the omelet in half and cut into three wedges. Repeat with other half of eggs. Serve omelets.

Egg pie

5 Servings

1 large sweet potato (grated)

1 tbsp. coconut oil (melted)

8 eggs

1 c. veggies (roasted)

4 strips cooked bacon (chopped)

1 tsp. sausage seasoning

Apply a thin layer of coconut oil of pie plate and mix sweet potato. Press down to the bottom & sides of the pie plate. Sprinkle some salt and pepper. Bake in oven at 350 to 375 degree for 20 minutes. Take out sweet potato's crust from oven. Sprinkle veggies in the base of plate and sausage seasoning over veggies. Break the eggs on top of veggies equally over the whole pie crust. Sprinkle bacon on the top and again bake in oven at 350 degree for 15 minutes or until eggs cooked as desired.

Carrot Banana Muffins

6-8 Servings

2 cup almond flour (blanched)

2 tsp. baking soda

1 tsp. Celtic sea salt

1 tbsp. cinnamon

1 cup dates (pitted)

3 bananas

3 eggs

1 tsp. apple cider vinegar

14 cup coconut oil (melted)

1 ½ cup carrots (shredded)

3/4 cup walnuts (finely chopped)

Take a small bowl and combine almond flour, salt, baking soda and cinnamon. Add dates, bananas, eggs, vinegar and oil in a food processor and mix well, set aside the mixture in a large bowl. Add dry mixture into wet and thoroughly combine it. Sprinkle in carrots and walnuts, spoon mixture into paper lined muffin pans. Bake it at 350 degrees up to 25 minutes and serve hot.

Paleo Breakfast Bars

6-8 Servings

1 c. almond flour (lightened)

1/4 c. coconut oil

1/4 tsp. Celtic sea salt

1/2 c. unsweetened coconut (shredded)

1/2 c. pumpkin seeds

1/2 c. sunflower seeds

1/4 c. slivered almonds (lightened)

1/4 c. raisins

2 tbsp. honey

1 tbsp. water

1 tsp. vanilla extract

Take a food processor, add all the ingredients and pulse in (mix) well. Press dough into an 8x8 inch baking dish. Wet your hands with water to press the dough down. Now, bake it at 350 degrees for 20 minutes. Cool down the bars in the pan for 2 hours before serving.

Lunch

Quick Red and Green Salsa

2 Servings

1 c. tomatoes (chopped)

1 red chili (seeded & diced)

1/2 mild green chili (seeded & diced)

2 tbsp. balsamic vinegar

1 tbsp. fresh chives (chopped)

1 tbsp. fresh cilantro (chopped)

Salt (to taste)

Take a bowl and combine all the ingredients. Serve as a dip or seasoning.

4 Servings

1 lb. chicken boneless breasts

16 oz. salsa verde

1/3 cup sundried tomatoes

2 cloves garlic

2 tbsp. olive oil

2 tbsp. balsamic vinegar

Slice the chicken into small pieces. Add tomatoes, garlic, olive oil and vinegar in a saucepan and Sauté until tender. Now put in chicken & cook until ready. Put salsa in saucepan and cook for 5 minutes. Serve chicken topped with salsa.

Paleo Salmon Sesame Seed Salad

4-6 Servings

3 oz. salmon (grilled)

8 asparagus

3 cherry tomatoes (sliced)

1/4 c. baby spinach (cleaned)

2 tbsp. sesame seeds

1 tbsp. coconut oil or olive oil

Take a saucepan and add coconut oil or olive oil. Sauté salmon & season to taste, cook until thoroughly cooked and set aside. Now cook asparagus until tender, set aside. Lay baby spinach over salad dishes and cover with spinach, salmon, tomatoes and asparagus. Coat with sesame seeds and serve.

Chili Beef Casserole

6 Servings

1/2 lb. lean ground beef

10 3/4 ounce tomato soup (undiluted)

1/2 tsp. chili powder

1/4 tsp. salt

1/4 tsp. pepper

6 green onions (chopped)

2.25 ounce sliced ripe olives (drained)

Take a large skillet and cook ground beef, stir until crumbles. Add tomato soup, chili powder, salt and pepper and cook on medium heat for 8 to 10 minutes, keep stirring occasionally. Lightly grease an 11 x 7 inch baking dish and add the meat mixture them top with green onion and olives. Bake it in oven uncovered at 350 degrees for 20 minutes or until ready. Sprinkle with additional green onion and serve.

Low-Fat Baked Crabmeat

8 Servings

1 c. sweet red pepper or green pepper (chopped)

1/2 c. celery (chopped)

2 tbsp. fresh parsley (chopped)

1 tsp. prepared mustard

1/8 tsp. freshly ground pepper

1/8 tsp. hot sauce

 2 large eggs

1/3 c. Paleo mayonnaise (calorie reduced)

1/3 c. fresh crabmeat (drained & flaked)

Olive oil

Take a nonstick skillet and coat with olive oil. Place it over medium high heat until hot; add pepper and celery and sauté for 5 minutes or until tender. Remove from heat and add parsley, ground pepper, mustard, hot sauce and stir well. Take another bowl and beat eggs lightly and mix with mayonnaise. Stir until smooth. Put in celery mixture & crabmeat, stir softly. Put in it in baking cups and place on baking sheet. Bake in oven at 375 degrees for 15 to 20 minutes.

Mexican Shellfish Stew

4 Servings

250 g. chicken stock

2 c. clam broth (fresh fish stock)

2 large any chilies (seeded)

3 medium garlic cloves (peeled)

8 oz. Tomatoes (drained)

2 tbsp. olive oil

20 small clams (scrubbed)

3/4 lb. medium shrimp (peeled & deveined)

1 small onion (minced)

2 tbsp. cilantro (minced)

Take a soup kettle and bring the chicken stock and the clam broth to boil. Add the chilies and simmer until softened for 10 minutes. Drain the chilies and set aside the cooking liquid. Take a food processor and add chilies, 1/3 cup cooking liquid, garlic, tomatoes and process until smooth. Strain puréed chili mixture through a fine strainer into a bowl and discard the solids. Now heat olive oil in the soup kettle, add purée juice and cook on medium heat, keep stirring for about 5 minutes or until this mixture gets slightly thickened. Put in the reserved chili cooking liquid and bring it boil. Put in clams and shrimp and simmer until the clams open and the shrimp gets opaque for 3 minutes. Scoop the soup and a portion of the clams and the shrimp into soup bowls. Shake over of each bowl with minced onions and cilantro and serve.

Mexican styled chorizo

6-8 Servings

1kg. finely chopped pork shoulder

500g finely chopped pork belly

30 g. sea salt

25 g. ground sweet paprika

25 g. ground smoked paprika

2 tsp. ground cayenne pepper

4 cloves of garlic finely minced

Some fennel seeds

2 tsp. pepper

4 oz. red wine

Take a large bowl, combine all the ingredients and mix thoroughly using your hands. Transfer it into a plastic bowl, cover and place in the fridge for 24 hours. Pour off any of the salty liquid from the bowl and add extra salt to taste. Keep in the fridge for a couple of hours. Take out the bowl and make patties from the mixture. Sauté for 5 minutes over medium heat. Then turn up the heat and add to the pan the scallops. They need about a 1 minute on each side. Combine, the seared scallops and chorizo onto the mixed salad leaves and serve.

Bacon Avocado Burritos

8 Servings

4 eggs

8 Paleo flour tortillas (7")

2 tbsp. olive oil

1 large avocado (thinly sliced)

1½ cup green onions (chopped)

1 lb. sliced bacon (cooked & crumbled)

Salsa

Take a large skillet, add oil and warm on medium high heat. Take a shallow bowl and beat eggs. Dip tortilla one by one in eggs and cook in oil on both sides just until egg sets. Take out and put on paper towels to drain, keep warm. Lay avocado, onions & bacon in the middle of tortillas. Put salsa on top. Fold its ends & sides over filling, roll up. Store or serve warm if desired.

Paleo Mexican Chop Salad

4 Servings

3 c. romaine lettuce (shredded)

2 c. red cabbage (shredded)

1/2 c. red onion (diced)

1 c. tomato (diced)

2 c. cucumbers (diced)

1/2 c. cilantro (chopped)

1 avocado (cubed)

1/2 c. sunflower seeds (toasted)

Ingredients for Salad Dressing

3 tbsp. orange juice

3 tbsp. apple cider vinegar

1 ½ Sea salt

1 tbsp. honey

1/2 cup olive oil

3/4 tsp. chili powder

Slice or shred lettuce and red cabbage in a food processor. Transfer it to a large bowl. Add diced tomato, red onion, cucumbers, cilantro, and avocado. Combine all salad dressing ingredients together. Combine the dressing in the bowl mixture. Serve with top toasted sunflower seeds.

Dinner

Blackened Tilapia and Mango Salsa

4 Serving

For Blackened Tilapia

3 tbsp. paprika

1 tbsp. onion powder

1 pinch garlic powder

1 tsp. white pepper

1 tsp. ground black pepper

1 tsp. cayenne pepper (to taste)

1 tsp. dried oregano

1 tsp. dried thyme

1/2 tsp. celery seed

1 tbsp. salt (to taste)

1 lb. tilapia fillet

1 lemon (cut into wedges)

1 tbsp. olive oil

For Mango Salsa

1 c. ripe seeded tomatoes (roughly chopped)

1 c. mango (diced)

1/2 c. cilantro (finely diced)

1/2 c. red onion (finely diced)

1 tsp. garlic powder

1/2 tsp. of salt

1/2 tsp. black pepper

1 Serrano chili, finely diced (Remove seed & veins)

Take a small bowl and combine all spices. Coat the fish fillets with this spices mixture and allow it to sit at room temperature for no longer than 30 minutes. Now add oil in skillet and warm it on high heat. Cook fillets for about 3 minutes from each side or until fish is thick and can be flaked with a fork. Remove it from the pan, pour pan juices over them and squeeze lemon juice all over. For mango salsa, mix all ingredients and refrigerate overnight to enhance flavors. Serve with already ready fish fillets.

Mexican Salsa Verde

4 Servings

1/2 c. onion (chopped)

1/2 lb. green tomatillo (shell removed)

1/2 c. cilantro (chopped)

2 tbsp. lime juice

2 jalapeño peppers (seeded & chopped)

Salt and pepper (to taste)

Slice the tomatillos laterally and bake on the grill for about 6 minutes until a little dark. Take a blender or food processor and put in the roasted tomatillos, cilantro, lime juice onion and jalapeño. Blend it until completely processed. Chill well, before use and then serve.

Mexican Chicken and Rice

4 Servings

4 tbsp. olive oil

1 medium onion (diced)

1 c. celery (finely diced)

1 head cauliflower (trimmed)

4 oz. green chilies (diced)

1 lb. boneless chicken breast (grilled & diced into 1" pieces)

1 tsp. Celtic sea salt

1 avocado

Ground cumin, oregano & chili powder (to taste)

Salsa (optional)

Take a large skillet, add olive oil and heat over medium heat. Sauté onion on medium heat for 10 minutes or until soft, add celery and again sauté for 5 minutes. Slice cauliflower in food processor & process until the texture of rice. Put cauliflower into skillet, cover it and cook for 5 to 10 minutes or until soft. Mix up chicken and chilies into skillet, stir in salt, oregano, cumin and chili powder. Top with avocado / salsa and serve.

Sausage and Kale Sauté

3-4 Servings

1 lb. sausage

1 bunch organic kale

1 medium onion (diced)

1/2 red bell pepper (chopped)

Take a large saucepan and add sausage to cook until browned. Put in onion and continue cooking on medium heat until onion becomes soft. Remove the spike of the kale and slice into small pieces, add it into the saucepan. Stir and cook until it softens or turns to bright green for 5 to 10 minutes. Remove saucepan from the heat and whisk chopped red bell pepper. Serve it warm.

Chicken Tortilla Soup

6 Servings

425 g. whole kernel corn (drained)

825 g. chicken broth

285 g. chunk chicken

285 g. tomatoes (diced)

Green chili peppers (drained)

Take a large saucepan and combine all the ingredients. Simmer it over medium high heat until cooked. Serve it warm.

Spicy Paprika and Lime Chicken

5-6 Servings

900 g. chicken tenderloins

5 tsp. sweet paprika

1 tsp. cayenne pepper or chili powder

1 ½ tsp. Celtic salt or sea salt

1 tsp. black pepper

3 tbsp. olive oil

2 garlic cloves (finely chopped)

2 tsp. tomato paste

2 limes

Coconut oil (for frying)

Take a large bowl, mix all marinade ingredients. Cut the chicken in large pieces and make long slices. Add pieces in marinade bowl and pat with your hands, cover and set aside for 1 hour before grilling. Heat one tbsp. of coconut oil in a frying pan or a grill plate until sizzling hot. Sauté chicken pieces from both sides for 3 minutes; set aside. Put cooked chicken in serving plates and sprinkle with lime juice before serving.

Desserts and Snacks

Paleo Spiced Nuts

4 Servings

2/3 c. almonds

2/3 c. pecans

2/3 c. walnuts

1 tsp. chili powder

1/2 tsp. cumin

1/2 tsp. ground black pepper

1/2 tsp. Celtic sea salt

1 tbsp. olive oil

Take a large skillet, add almond, pecans & walnuts and warm over medium heat, toast until lightly browned. Combine all other spices in a small bowl. Add olive oil over and the coat with spices mixture.

Churro Rounds

4-6 Servings

2 c. almond flour (blanched)

1/8 tsp. Celtic sea salt

1/8 tsp. baking soda

1 tsp. cinnamon

1/4 c. vegan shortening

2 tbsp. honey

1/2 cup coconut sugar (for dipping)

1 tbsp. cinnamon (for dipping)

Take a food processor, mix almond flour, baking soda, salt, and cinnamon. Beat in the shortening and honey. Make balls from the dough by taking 1 tbsp. scoop from dough. Dip the balls in a small bowl of water and roll in to coat with coconut sugar and cinnamon. Place balls on parchment paper lined baking sheets and shape it flat with the hand. Bake it in oven at 350° for 7-9 minutes. Chill well before serving.

Paleo Vegetable Shake

3 Servings

2 c. fresh spinach

3 stalks fresh kale

1/2 c. fresh blueberries

1/2 large orange

1/2 c. coconut milk

2 bananas (peeled)

1 tbsp. ground flax seed

Honey (optional)

Wash all the fruits and vegetables. Take a blender, add kale, spinach and coconut milk and blend thoroughly. Now put in remaining ingredients and blend well. Chill and then serve.

Stuffed Cantaloupe with Blackberries & Pecans

2 Servings

1 cantaloupe

1 c. blackberries

1/2 c. pecans (chopped)

Mint or spearmint leaves (for garnish)

Slice cantaloupe in half. Scoop out seeds and fill each hollow space with blackberries and pecans.

Use mint or spearmint leaves to garnish & Serve.

Stuffed Cantaloupe with Blackberries & Pecans

Cherry Berry Medley

4 Servings

1/2 c. rainier cherries (pitted & chopped)

1/2 c. blueberries

1/2 c. golden raspberries

1/2 c. blackberries

1 tsp. vanilla extract

1/2 tsp. clove powder

1/2 tsp. cinnamon

1 fresh mint leave (chopped)

Mint leaves (for garnish)

Take a medium sized bowl and combine cherries and berries. Put in vanilla, cinnamon, clove, chopped mint and toss gently. Chill for 30 minutes and garnish with mint leaves before serving.

Lemon Lavender Cookies

4-6 Servings

1¼ c. almond flour (blanched)

1/4 tsp. Celtic sea salt

1/4 tsp. baking soda

2 tsp. dried lavender (finely minced)

1/4 c. grape seed oil

3 tbsp. agave nectar

1 tbsp. lemon zest

Take a large bowl and combine dry ingredients. In a smaller bowl, stir wet ingredients together. Now mix both the dry & wet ingredients and form 1/2 inch balls and press onto a parchment paper lined baking sheet. Bake in oven at 350° for 7 to 10 minutes. Cool it down and serve.

Mexican Chocolate Coffee Cake

4-6 Servings

6 eggs

1/2 c. coconut oil (melted)

1/2 c. coconut flour

1/3 c. cacao powder

3 oz. unsweetened chocolate (melted)

1/2 c. blackstrap molasses

1/2 c. honey

2 tsp. vanilla extract

1/2 tsp. salt

1/2 tsp. baking soda

1 tsp. ground cinnamon

1/2 tsp. cayenne pepper (to taste)

Pre-heat an oven to 325 degrees. Line 5 X 9 inch loaf pan with wax paper, grease wax paper with coconut oil. Take a small bowl and sift the cocoa, cinnamon, cayenne, coconut flour, salt and baking soda. Combine eggs, molasses, honey and vanilla in a food processor and pulse together. Put in coconut oil, chocolate and process / blend for 1 minute. Now add dry ingredients into it & pulse to combine. Transfer batter into ready loaf pan and bake for 50 to 60 minutes. Let it cool down completely in pan and remove the wax paper cautiously.